Friendship

The Power and Beauty of
of
Friendship

Jose Valladares

Contents

A Guide

• • • • • •

Scope of this book

"The Power and Beauty of Friendship" is an extensive exploration of friendship and its evolution into love. It provides a
multifaceted understanding of different types of friendships,
their dynamics, and the challenges they may face over time.
The book delves into how friendship can lead to deeper emotional connections, emphasizing the role of purity and value
in this transition. It provides practical strategies for fostering
strong bonds and maintaining enduring relationships, even
when dealing with difficulties. The book concludes by reflecting on the transformative power of love and friendship in our
lives. It's an invaluable resource for anyone seeking to enrich
their understanding of personal relationships and appreciate
the significance of friendship.

God is the Love that Became God

Introduction

In the grand tapestry of human existence, few threads are woven as consistently and profoundly as those of friendship. From the earliest days of communal living to the complex social dynamics of the modern world, friendship remains a vital part of our shared human experience. As we delve into this book, "The Power and Beauty of Friendship," we embark on an exploration of the delicate yet resilient bonds of camaraderie that define us as social beings.

In these pages, we delve into the multifaceted nature of friendship, drawing from philosophy, psychology, and our own personal narratives to illuminate the diverse aspects of this universal bond. We journey from the joyful companionship of reciprocal friendships to the complex dynamics of unequal bonds, exploring how these relationships shape us and are shaped by us.

We delve into the power of friendship – its capacity to uplift, to heal, to transform. Friendship is not merely a bond between individuals; it is a catalyst for personal growth, a mirror reflecting our virtues and flaws, a safety net offering solace and support in times of crisis. Friendship endows us with courage, emboldens us with confidence, and blesses us with a sense of belonging.

Equally, we immerse ourselves in the beauty of friendship – the comfort of shared memories, the solace of unconditional acceptance, the joy of mutual growth. We explore how the beauty of friendship extends beyond the realm of emotions, manifesting in actions, influences, and the societal structures that uphold and celebrate these invaluable connections.

Yet, our exploration goes further. We venture into the intersection of friendship and love, unveiling the ways these potent emotions intertwine and enhance one another. The lines between love and friendship often blur, each adding depth, strength, and richness to the other.

"The Power and Beauty of Friendship" is more than a celebration of camaraderie and companionship. It is a homage to the bonds that unite us, the shared experiences that define us, and the enduring love that sustains us. As you turn these pages, may you find insights that resonate with your own experiences, inspire new perspectives, and enhance your understanding and appreciation of the power and beauty of friendship.

Friendship often forms the foundational stone on the journey to love. When two individuals come together as friends, they establish a relationship based on shared interests, mutual respect, and a genuine understanding of each other's strengths and weaknesses. As this bond of friendship strengthens over time, it often gives rise to a deeper, more profound feeling of love. It is through the shared laughter, mutual support during hardships, and the joy of simply being together that friendship subtly and gradually metamorphoses into love.

However, it's important to remember that this evolution is not automatic or inevitable. It stems from the authentic appreciation of the other person as an individual, independent

God is the Love that Became God

of any ulterior motives or expectations. It is when we learn to value the other person for their unique qualities, their idiosyncrasies, their dreams, and even their flaws that friendship can develop into love. This transition, while not always seamless, is marked by a deepened understanding, an intensified connection, and an unwavering commitment to each other's well-being.

Purity in friendship plays an essential role in this transition. Pure friendship is characterized by selflessness, honesty, and a desire to contribute positively to the other person's life. It is not swayed by selfish motives, nor is it contingent on material or external conditions. When friendship is pure, it fosters a sense of security and trust that forms the bedrock of love.

Valuing purity in friendship implies appreciating and nurturing the core tenets of friendship, such as empathy, kindness, and mutual respect. It involves maintaining an atmosphere of openness and honesty, offering support without seeking anything in return, and cherishing the other person's happiness as our own. When these values are upheld, friendship transcends its conventional boundaries and becomes a transformative force, capable of leading to the path of love.

The importance of valuing purity in friendship cannot be overstated. It safeguards the bond from external influences, strengthens the connection, and allows the friendship to serve as a source of joy, comfort, and personal growth. It's through this purity that the deepest form of love – one that is patient, understanding, and enduring – can blossom. It's a love that sees beyond the superficial, embraces individuality, and values the essence of the person.

In conclusion, the journey from friendship to love is a beautiful and fulfilling path, guided by shared experiences, mutual respect, and a deep understanding of each other. The purity and value of friendship play an instrumental role in this transition, fostering a bond that can weather life's challenges and thrive in its joys. It is through this purity that love, in its most profound and meaningful form, emerges. Therefore, cherishing and nurturing the purity of friendship is not just important, but essential in allowing love to flourish.

Chapter 1

The Foundation of Connection

1.1 The Genesis of Bonds:

Understanding the Distinct Types of Friendship

When we study friendships, we discover a variety of relationships formed for different reasons. This leads us to classify friendships into three main types, each reflecting a unique kind of affection where friends sincerely care for each other's welfare.

The first type is a "friendship of utility". Here, individuals become friends due to the benefits they receive from each other. For instance, this could be friends in a business context who help each other succeed in their respective careers. It's important to note, however, that in these friendships, people like each other primarily for the benefits they provide, not necessarily for their individual personalities.

The second type is a "friendship of pleasure". In this case, friends are drawn to each other because they find each other's company enjoyable. This might be a group of friends who meet weekly to play board games or enjoy hiking together. But like the first type, the affection here is conditional, dependent on the shared activity or the fun derived from the interaction. If the enjoyable aspects disappear, these friendships may dissolve.

The third and deepest form of friendship is a "friendship of virtue". This friendship is based on mutual admiration for each other's character and values. For example, this might be two friends who share a passion for volunteering and giving back to their community. They genuinely care about each other's happiness and well-being, beyond their own self-interest. This type of friendship is fulfilling, long-lasting, and often the most satisfying.

While friendships of utility and pleasure play certain roles in our lives, they are often less stable and satisfying than friendships of virtue. A friendship based on utility may end when the usefulness decreases. Similarly, a friendship based on pleasure might cease to exist as personal tastes evolve. However, a friendship based on virtue is more resilient because it's anchored in shared values and moral appreciation, providing a deep connection and personal growth.

However, it's also important to understand that friendships of virtue are less common and take longer to develop. They require mutual understanding, trust, and acknowledgement of each other's character. It's through shared experiences, overcoming challenges, and the gradual growth of trust that these bonds of friendship mature. While casual acquaintanceship is common, a true and deep friendship is a lifelong bond that recognizes the inherent worth in each other and a commitment to each other's well-being.

In essence, friendship takes many forms, each with its own purpose. Although friendships of utility and pleasure have their places in our lives, it's the friendships of virtue that truly motivate and uplift us. These friendships, characterized

God is the Love that Became God

by genuine care, shared values, and a mutual desire for each other's success, provide us with joy, support, and a deep sense of belonging. As we navigate life, let's treasure and nurture these profound friendships, as they have the power to infuse our lives with love and immeasurable enrichment.

1.2 Deep Bonds and Goodness:
The Roots of Companionship

Friendship, a manifestation of virtuous behavior or a reflection of virtuous qualities, is pivotal in leading a wholesome and fulfilling life. The significance of friendship extends beyond material possessions and wealth. Individuals, even those with abundant resources or elevated positions of power, can lead a life devoid of joy and meaning without the presence of genuine friends. Moreover, people in such privileged positions often have a heightened need for friendships. After all, wealth and prosperity serve their purpose best when they offer opportunities to extend kindness and generosity, notably towards friends.

Friends act as guardians and stewards of our well-being and prosperity. As our successes increase, so does our vulnerability to potential risks and adversities. In times of poverty or hardship, friends often become our sanctuary, offering emotional solace and consolation. For the younger demographic, friendships serve as guiding lights, helping them to circumvent mistakes and offering a sense of direction. For the elderly, friends step in to lend assistance, filling the void left by declining abilities. During the prime of life, friendships motivate noble endeavors and foster deep introspection and meaningful action.

A closer look at the animal kingdom reveals that bonds akin to friendship are not unique to humans. The connection between parents and offspring is observed in numerous species, including birds. Such natural camaraderie among beings of the same species emphasizes the fundamental importance of friendship. Society, as a whole, praises individuals who display affection and care for others. It's crucial to recognize that each person we encounter, in our journeys, holds their own unique significance.

Friendship serves as the unifying force in communities, often considered paramount even over the rigorous enforcement of justice. Genuine friendships reduce the necessity for excessive legal interventions, as they embody a sense of fairness and mutual respect. When individuals seek justice, they naturally gravitate towards the companionship and support of their friends, thereby weaving friendship and justice inextricably together.

In summary, friendship is not only essential but inherently noble. An individual with a multitude of friends is admired as it mirrors their goodness and capacity to foster meaningful relationships. Opinions about the nature of friendship vary, with some arguing that true friendship is born out of similarity - as captured by the saying "like attracts like". Conversely, others suggest that individuals with similar interests or professions may not necessarily harmonize. Various theories draw parallels with natural phenomena or propose that opposing forces can result in mutual benefits, to further dissect the complexities of friendship. These explorations encourage us to delve deeper into the nature of friendship. They pose intriguing questions such as whether anyone is capable of forming genuine friendships, whether individuals with wicked tendencies can establish true friendships, and whether there exists one or multiple forms of friendship. These themes have been discussed in-depth in previous conversations and offer valuable insights into the multifaceted concept of friendship.

1.3 The Power of True Friendship:
An Unseen Force

Within the varied landscape of human relationships, friendship stands out as a unique bond that adds immense value to our lives. Among the diverse types of friendships, there is one kind that outshines the rest in its depth, longevity, and the mutual benefit it offers. This is the friendship rooted in goodness. Let's delve deeper into the characteristics of this special bond and how it nurtures love.

In this exceptional form of friendship, the friends share a profound connection and understanding. They engage in a reciprocal exchange that fosters a deep sense of harmony and mutual support. Both friends benefit from each other equally, or at least in ways that bring about comparable outcomes. This is what makes this type of friendship ideal and perfect, representing the quintessence of a balanced relationship between friends.

Another form of friendship, which aligns with this perfect form, is the friendship of pleasure. When individuals of good character come together, their shared experiences often lead to joy and delight. The pleasure they derive from each other's company naturally enhances the warmth and strength of their friendship. Similarly, friendship based on utility can also be closely associated with the perfect form. Good people often find each other useful, which further strengthens their bond.

In contrast, friendships rooted solely in pleasure or utility tend to lack the same depth and resilience. While these friendships can endure when both friends derive the same thing from each other, they differ from relationships such as romantic ones, where one person might take pleasure in just seeing their partner, while the other seeks attention and affection. As time passes and the initial passion fades, these friendships may dissolve if the source of pleasure diminishes. However, in some cases, the bond evolves and survives based on an appreciation of each other's character and the familiarity that develops over time.

Friendships based on utility are generally less authentic and less enduring. When the usefulness of the friendship ceases, the bond often dissolves, revealing that the affection was more for the benefit provided than for the person themselves. Thus, friendships centered on personal pleasure or utility lack the depth and lasting power of those grounded in goodness and mutual benefit.

True friendships, formed on the bedrock of mutual benefit and goodness, are enduring and resistant to slander and doubts. In these relationships, both friends are of good character, having earned each other's trust over time. Trust is a fundamental element of such friendships, which leaves no room for doubts or rumors. Believing that "my friend would never wrong me" and having faith in each other's character are typical of friendships between good people. In contrast, friendships rooted in pleasure or utility are more vulnerable to these challenges, as they lack the foundation of inherent goodness that fosters mutual trust and respect.

It's worth mentioning that relationships formed for pleasure or utility are often loosely referred to as friendships. An analogy can be drawn with the alliances between nations, which are seen as friendly due to their mutual benefits. Similarly, relationships based on shared pleasure, such as those among children, are also labeled as friendships. However, while these relationships might share certain traits with genuine friendship, they are not the same. They lack the depth, resilience, and profound connection characteristic of true friendships.

Genuine friendship is a potent force that fosters meaningful bonds between people. It is a relationship rooted in goodness and mutual benefit, characterized by a deep sense of understanding and connection. This special form of friendship surpasses all others in its resilience and capacity to nurture love. As we navigate our relationships in life, it's important to recognize the value of true friendship and invest time and effort in nurturing such bonds.

Chapter 2

The Dynamics of Friendship

2.1 The Beauty of Unequal Friendship:
A Different Perspective

Alongside the more traditional forms of friendship, there lies a unique variant that flourishes despite, or perhaps because of, the inherent inequality between the individuals involved. These unequal friendships, such as those between a parent and child or a ruler and subject, exhibit unique attributes and dynamics. While these relationships might involve love and friendship, it's essential to understand that these experiences are not identical across different relationships. The virtues, roles, and motivations that drive the love in these relationships vary, shaping the nature of the bond.

In unequal friendships, each individual does not expect the same from the other, nor should they aim for such parity. A parent doesn't seek the same things from their child as the child seeks from the parent, for instance. However, when individuals fulfill their respective responsibilities — such as children respecting their parents and parents caring for their children — a deep and enduring friendship can blossom. In these relationships marked by inherent inequality, the expression of love should be proportional. The person who sur-

God is the Love that Became God

passes the other in virtue or usefulness should be loved more than they love in return. It's this principle of proportionality that introduces a form of equality into these relationships, a fundamental characteristic of genuine friendship.

Yet, it's important to underscore that equality manifests differently in the domains of justice and friendship. In the pursuit of justice, the primary focus is on proportional equality, reflecting the merit of each person, while quantitative equality plays a secondary role. In friendship, however, the emphasis shifts. Quantitative equality becomes more significant, while proportional equality becomes less so. This distinction becomes apparent when the gap in virtue, vice, wealth, or other factors between the parties is substantial. When this disparity grows too wide, the individuals may no longer regard each other as friends and may not expect to maintain the friendship. A clear illustration of this is the divine realm, where gods far exceed humans in every aspect, making the notion of friendship between them implausible. Similarly, subjects do not usually anticipate friendships with kings, and individuals of modest means do not foresee friendships with those of exceptional wisdom or wealth. Identifying the exact bounds of friendship under these circumstances can be challenging. While minor differences can exist without rupturing the bond, when one party far outstrips the other — as in the case of gods compared to humans — the likelihood of friendship diminishes significantly.

This raises a philosophical question about the nature of friendship. If friends genuinely desire the best for each other — such as achieving divinity — wouldn't such a transformation ultimately dissolve the friendship? This is because the resulting inequality would render the friendship irrelevant and non-beneficial. The solution to this conundrum lies in the idea that friends wish for their friends' wellbeing for their friends' sake. Consequently, a friend should wish for their friend to remain as they are, retaining their essential nature, including their humanity. Therefore, in friendships, people primarily desire for their friends the greatest goods that are compatible with their friends' human nature. They might not necessarily desire every conceivable good, such as achieving godlike status.

Unequal friendships thus represent a celebration of diversity, and an acknowledgement that love and friendship can thrive amidst differences in status, virtue, or roles. Through proportionality and acceptance of inherent limitations, these relationships can nurture genuine connections, fostering deep love and understanding. These friendships underscore the multiplicity of human bonds and the nuanced ways in which we connect, care for, and value each other.

2.2 Connection, Character & Equality:

The Trifecta of Friendship

Friendship is a profoundly significant aspect of our lives, serving as a fertile ground for deep bonds of love and connection. It's important to understand that the essence of friendship is not confined to mere physical proximity. Friendship is enriched by shared activities and mutual benefit, yet it extends beyond simply living together or being in the same place. Even when distance separates friends or when time apart interrupts the habitual activities of friendship, the core bond remains. It is deeply rooted in our shared disposition, our mutual understanding, and our desire to partake in acts of friendship. Although distance might temporarily pause the tangible expressions of friendship, it doesn't nullify the bond. However, extended periods of separation can test the resilience of friendship, leading to the forgetting of the shared closeness, as the saying goes, "out of sight, out of mind."

Forming friendships can pose challenges for older individuals or those who have a disagreeable or sour demeanor. If a person lacks pleasantness, it's harder for others to enjoy their company. Spending time with someone who's not enjoyable or who elicits discomfort is naturally undesirable. Guided by natural instincts, we're drawn towards companionship that brings us happiness and fulfillment. Our innate pursuit of pleasure and avoidance of pain steer us towards forging bonds with those who offer pleasant experiences and add joy to our lives. It's crucial to distinguish between individuals who enjoy each other's company but do not live together, and those who share a deep bond of true friendship. The former may harbor goodwill towards each other, while the latter enjoys a bond enriched by shared experiences and compatibility. True friendship blooms through living together, sharing life's journey, and resonating with each other.

The most admirable form of friendship is found among virtuous individuals. Such friendships transcend superficial connections and are steeped in goodness and pleasantness. Goodness and pleasantness are intrinsically lovable and desirable qualities, not only in a broad sense but also on a personal level. When two virtuous individuals become friends, their shared goodness uplifts both their own lives and each other's. Love, in this context, is not a fleeting emotion but rather a reflection of their character. Friendship arises from a deeply rooted state of character, where individuals voluntarily choose to prioritize the well-being and happiness of their friends. Within this bond, love and friendship interweave, giving rise to a reciprocal exchange of goodwill and pleasant experiences. Friendship at its core rests on the principles of equality, where both parties give and receive in equitable measure. The friendship of virtuous individuals exemplifies these traits to the highest degree, forging a profound and enduring connection based on mutual respect, shared values, and genuine love.

As we journey through life, it's important to treasure and nurture true friendship. This remarkable bond enriches our lives, fills our hearts with joy, and serves as a reminder of the inherent goodness within us and those around us. A bond that, even when tested by distance or time, remains resilient, reminding us of our shared humanity and mutual love.

2.3 The Nuances of Friendship:

Exploring the Subtleties

In the realm of friendship, not all individuals have an equal propensity for forming deep connections. Certain individuals, particularly those of a sour disposition or older age, may encounter difficulties in cultivating friendships. This is often due to their less amicable nature and diminished capacity to enjoy social interactions, two crucial elements that underpin the foundation of friendship. Friendship flourishes in an environment of mutual pleasure and amicability, which are indispensable for the formation of deep and lasting bonds. Consequently, older and less affable individuals may find it challenging to quickly establish close connections. While they may bear goodwill towards one another and can offer help during times of need, the lack of shared enjoyable experiences and mutual pleasure prevents them from truly encapsulating the essence of friendship.

In the pursuit of genuine, pure friendships, one cannot successfully extend such connections to a multitude of people simultaneously. Similar to how it is untenable to be romantically involved with multiple people at the same time, authentic friendship demands an intense and exclusive bond. To truly please and feel appreciated by one person necessitates an intricate interplay of understanding, familiarity, and mutual respect. This level of connection proves challenging to achieve when diluted across multiple relationships. However, it is more feasible in friendships based on utility or pleasure, as these types require less depth and are often established for the mutual benefit or enjoyment they bring, rather than for their own sake.

Among these secondary types of friendships, those formed for the sake of pleasure are most akin to authentic friendships. In these relationships, the parties derive joy from each other's company and from their shared activities. Acts of generosity and goodwill are common, providing a sense of enjoyment that strengthens the bond. In contrast, friendships based on utility are generally more pragmatic, revolving around the benefits that each party can provide. Individuals in positions of authority often have a spectrum of friends: some are there for their utility, and others for the pleasure they provide. However, finding an individual who encapsulates both usefulness and pleasantness is a rare occurrence.

While friendships based on pleasure and utility may exhibit characteristics similar to genuine friendship, significant differences remain. A virtuous friendship is a friendship of the highest order, encompassing not only mutual pleasure and utility but also a deep appreciation of the friend's character for its own sake. It thrives on the principles of reciprocity and equality, where the friends mirror each other's feelings and share common desires. Conversely, friendships based on pleasure or utility lack the enduring and stable nature of authentic friendship. Although they contain certain elements of friendship, their lack of permanence and susceptibility to fluctuations in circumstances or feelings mark them as fundamentally different from friendships of virtue. While they share some characteristics with genuine friendships, their unique features and the relative lack of stability and resilience set them apart. Their status as genuine friendships thus remains open to question.

Chapter 3

The Inseparable Duo:

3.1 The True Nature of Love and Friendship:
A Close Examination

In the intricate web of human relationships, it's crucial to understand that many people are motivated more by a desire to be loved than by the wish to love others. This inclination often springs from an underlying ambition, leading individuals to value the admiration and affection they receive more than the sentiments they extend. Consequently, flattery becomes an attractive tool, as flatterers can masquerade as friends, seemingly loving more than they are loved. This craving for affection often intertwines with the desire for honor and recognition. Many people find solace in esteem and respect, as these confer a sense of validation and accomplishment. It's essential, however, to discern whether the pursuit of honor stems from an authentic aspiration or merely serves as a means to an end. Often, people derive satisfaction from being honored by those in positions of authority, not because of the honor itself, but because of the potential benefits they anticipate. They view the accolades they receive as harbingers of future advantages.

Contrasting this desire for honor, the joy derived from being loved is an intrinsically rewarding experience. This implies that being loved holds more profound value than merely being honored, highlighting the inherent desirability of genuine friendship. Notably, the crux of friendship doesn't lie in being loved, but in loving others. This truth is embodied in the unwavering love that mothers have for their children. Even in situations where mothers choose to have their children raised by others, their love endures as long as they are aware of their children's wellbeing. These mothers don't seek reciprocation of love; instead, they find fulfillment in seeing their children thrive, underlining the importance of love as a key ingredient in friendship and enduring bonds.

Furthermore, the essence of friendship is better understood through the act of loving rather than being loved. Genuine friendship stems from sincere care and affection, manifested in the love we extend to others. Those who embody this quality, with the right measure, can build lasting and meaningful friendships. This is particularly apparent when individuals share similar virtues, demonstrating steadfastness, integrity, and commitment to each other's well-being. True friends neither seek personal gain nor resort to selfish acts; instead, they actively deter each other from destructive paths. In contrast, friendships based solely on utility or pleasure typically last only as long as they provide mutual benefits or enjoyment. Relationships based on utility, such as those between the wealthy and the poor or the knowledgeable and the ignorant, revolve around the exchange of goods or services that meet specific needs. Likewise, friendships driven by pleasure, such as romantic relationships or bonds based on physical attractiveness, may dissolve if the pleasure fades or shared interests wane.

In the quest to foster love and friendship, we must shift our focus from a desire to be loved to the active extension of love to others. While the pursuit of honor can seem enticing, it is the inherent joy of being loved and the act of loving that truly enrich our souls. Genuine friendships are built on a foundation of mutual care, affection, and virtue. The essence of friendship lies not in the love we receive, but in the love we offer. By nurturing love and cultivating deep connections, we can experience the profound beauty and fulfillment that come from meaningful relationships.

3.2 Bonds of Love and the Essence of Emotional Connections:

A Deep Dive

Understanding the various dimensions of friendship necessitates examining the core essence of love. Love is not indiscriminate; rather, it is directed towards what one considers lovable. This lovable attribute is generally characterized by goodness, pleasantness, or usefulness. When something invokes a sense of goodness or pleasure, or serves a particular purpose, it becomes worthy of love, rendering goodness and usefulness intrinsically lovable.

When scrutinizing this concept further, one might question whether individuals primarily love what is objectively good or what is personally beneficial to them. These two perspectives can sometimes contradict, and a similar tension emerges in regards to what is deemed pleasant. Generally, people tend to love what they perceive as being good for them, irrespective of its objective value. The unqualified notion of goodness is universally deemed lovable. Even when this idea diverges from an objective standard, each person tends to regard what they consider personally beneficial as lovable. This differentiation, however, does not detract from the central theme; we can alternatively refer to this concept as "that which appears lovable."

Love arises from three key motivations: goodness, pleasantness, and usefulness. When discussing inanimate objects, we do not apply the term "friendship" because these objects lack the capacity for mutual affection and a genuine concern for the other party's well-being. For instance, it would be nonsensical to wish well to an inanimate object, such as a bottle of wine. However, in the context of friends, the notion of wishing genuine goodness for the other person is vital. If this mutual wish is not reciprocated, the relationship is attributed with goodwill rather than friendship. Yet, when both parties express a sincere desire for the other's well-being, their bond can accurately be termed as friendship.

This analysis brings us to a critical question: is mutual recognition a prerequisite for friendship? It's noteworthy that many people harbor goodwill towards those whom they have never met, based on their perception of these individuals as being good or useful. In some cases, this sentiment may be reciprocated, creating a mutual expression of goodwill. But can we truthfully label these individuals as friends if they remain unaware of the other's sentiments? A genuine friendship requires not just the mutual expression of goodwill, but also the recognition of it. The individuals involved must sincerely wish for each other's well-being, motivated by either goodness, pleasantness, or usefulness. The acknowledgment

God is the Love that Became God

of this mutual sentiment forms the bedrock of a true friendship.

3.3 Love through Friendship and Justice:
The Harmony of Affection and Fairness

Central to our exploration are the intertwined themes of
friendship and justice, both of which fundamentally influence our collective existence. These themes are intercon-
nected, revolving around shared interests and mutual bonds
among individuals. In every community, whether it's a society, a group of fellow travelers, or comrades in arms, we
observe the presence of justice and friendship. The strength
of these bonds is determined by our level of association with
others, indicative of the prevalence of justice in our interactions.

The age-old adage, "what friends have is common property," underscores the critical role that shared experiences
and possessions play in cultivating friendships. Siblings and
comrades share a profound sense of unity and commonality,
while other types of friendships may involve varying degrees of shared interests and possessions. Friendships come
in different forms and depths; some are more authentic and
profound than others. Similarly, the obligations and responsibilities of justice differ across various relationships. The
duties of parents towards their children differ from those of
siblings towards each other, just as comrades' responsibilities
differ from those of fellow citizens. These differences extend
to other types of friendships as well. Consequently, acts of

injustice hold different degrees of severity depending on the relationship's nature. A deceptive act against a comrade is viewed as more severe than against a fellow citizen, just as failing to assist a sibling is considered more significant than neglecting a stranger. Causing harm to a parent is deemed far graver than causing harm to another person. It suggests that the demands of justice intensify proportionally with the depth and strength of the friendship, indicating an inherent interplay between the two concepts.

Moreover, the essence of community transcends individual relationships to embrace a broader interconnectedness concept. All forms of community, borne out of practical needs or shared interests, are analogous to integral elements of the political community. Within these smaller communities, people come together in pursuit of specific advantages and to fulfill their needs. The political community, encompassing society at large, is built on the pursuit of collective benefits. Legislators and leaders work towards establishing a system that promotes the common good, making decisions that are considered beneficial for the community as a whole. While other communities might focus on specific advantages - such as sailors seeking profits from their voyages or soldiers seeking victory and wealth - they ultimately contribute to the broader objectives of the political community. Communities may also form from the pursuit of pleasure, seen in religious guilds and social clubs, focusing on religious offerings or fostering camaraderie, respectively. However, these diverse communities find their place within the political community, which covers long-term advantages and overall societal well-being. Rituals, gatherings, acts of devotion, and recreational activities serve as expressions of communal unity,

God is the Love that Became God

providing platforms for people to connect, strengthen their bonds, and create a sense of shared enjoyment and purpose. Thus, all communities, regardless of their specific objectives, contribute to the larger fabric of the political community, with different types of friendships aligning accordingly.

In the interplay of friendship and justice, we find the seeds of love woven into our communal existence. The bonds we form based on mutual care, shared experiences, and a sense of fairness, engender a profound sense of connection and belonging. As we navigate the intricacies of our communities, we must embrace the transformative power of friendship and justice, fostering a love that surpasses boundaries and instills harmony among us all.

Chapter 4

The Power and Influence of Love

4.1 The Power of Love in Various Forms of

Relationships:

A Broad View

Love is a powerful force that not only suffuses personal relationships but also infiltrates political systems. By investigating different constitutional types and their analogues in various relationships, we can gain a deeper understanding of love's extensive influence and its integral role in promoting unity and well-being.

In the sphere of political systems, there are three main forms of constitution: monarchy, aristocracy, and timocracy (also referred to as polity). These forms mirror diverse power dynamics and distributions of authority. Monarchy epitomizes the ideal form, where a king reigns with his subjects' welfare at the heart of his rule. It symbolizes the love and care a father holds for his children, cultivating a harmonious and nurturing environment. The relationship between a father and his children exemplifies the power of love in creating a just and thriving society.

However, monarchy can become distorted. Tyranny, the corrupt version of monarchy, takes hold when a ruler becomes egocentric, pursuing personal interests. This form of governance is devoid of love and empathy, leading to suppression and suffering. It acts as a stark reminder of the destructive nature of power devoid of love.

Aristocracy, characterized by the rule of a virtuous and deserving few, can degrade into oligarchy. In an aristocracy, the ruling class demonstrates love and goodwill towards their fellow citizens. They prioritize the communal good and act as custodians of justice. However, when the rulers in an aristocracy turn corrupt and selfish, the system mutates into an oligarchy. Love and unity are supplanted by avarice and inequality.

Timocracy, grounded on property qualifications, has the potential to devolve into democracy. Timocracy mirrors the love and respect shared among siblings, who consider each other as equals. But if significant disparities in wealth or power emerge, the system may veer into democracy, where decisions are collectively made and individual freedoms are emphasized. Democracy, albeit flawed, upholds the principles of equality and freedom, highlighting love's inclusive and egalitarian facets.

By scrutinizing these constitutional variations and their manifestations in personal relationships, we can perceive love's transformative capacity in engendering harmony, justice, and well-being. Love, when fostered and expressed in governance and personal connections, can engender a society grounded in compassion, fairness, and mutual respect. It's through the cultivation of love and empathy that we can instill a profound sense of connection, fostering a harmonious and inclusive world for all.

4.2 Nurturing Love:

Fostering Growth in Relationships

Friendship bears an impressive capacity to cultivate love, nurture profound connections, and engender camaraderie in diverse contexts. Whether manifested within familial ties, political structures, or societal interactions, the essence of friendship resonates deeply.

Within the realm of familial relations, the bond between a king and his subjects encapsulates the power of friendship that is rooted in acts of benevolence and kindness. A king, fueled by sincere concern for his subjects' well-being, emerges as a shepherd of his people, extending support, guidance, and protection. This nurturing friendship emerges from a deep-seated love that surpasses self-interest, reminiscent of the harmonious relationship between a shepherd and his flock.

Similarly, the bond between a father and his children illustrates friendship's immense potential to transcend boundaries. A father's love not only encapsulates the gift of life but also encompasses the responsibility of nurturing and guiding his offspring. This unconditional love and commitment lay the groundwork for a deep-rooted friendship, fostering a sense of belonging and trust within the family unit.

In the context of political structures, friendship also plays a significant role. Within an aristocracy, where individuals earn recognition and respect based on their virtue and excellence, the relationship between the ruler and the ruled evolves into a friendship steeped in mutual respect and shared objectives. A virtuous ruler prioritizes their subjects' well-being and strives to govern in a way that is beneficial to all, engendering unity, harmony, and love for the common good.

These contexts underscore the intimate connection between friendship and justice. The tenet of justice ensures fairness and equity in the distribution of benefits and responsibilities, thereby strengthening the bonds of friendship. Inherent in friendship is the reciprocity of care, support, and consideration, manifest in the relationships between rulers and subjects, parents and children, and those in positions of authority.

Moreover, friendship's influence extends beyond familial and political scenarios to include societal interactions. Whether it be in the companionship of siblings or the camaraderie of friends, the power of friendship remains potent. Siblings, bound by familial ties and shared experiences, foster a bond rooted in love, loyalty, and mutual understanding. Similarly, friendships among peers cultivate an atmosphere of shared values, support, and acceptance, reinforcing a sense of love and belonging.

However, it's important to note that friendship can be challenged in various forms of governance. For instance, tyranny hinders the formation of friendships as the ruler's self-interest trumps the welfare of their subjects. In such instances, love and camaraderie are stifled, and justice is undermined. Conversely, democratic systems, where equality is paramount, provide a nurturing environment for the growth of friendships and the flourishing of love, as individuals find common interests and shared aspirations.

In conclusion, friendship wields remarkable power to instill love and nurture deep connections across various spheres of life. From familial ties to political structures and societal interactions, the essence of friendship permeates, fostering a sense of belonging, trust, and mutual support. It's through the reciprocity of care, acts of kindness, and shared values that love flourishes, fortifying the bonds of friendship and enriching the human experience.

4.3 Love and Friendship in Various Relationships:

A Comparative Analysis

Love and friendship are fundamental to human connections, playing a pivotal role in various relationships. The exploration of these relationships and the nature of love and friendship within them can provide us with a richer understanding and appreciation of the bonds we share.

Kinship: The love that exists between family members, such as between parents and their children, represents a unique and deep form of friendship. Parents love their children unconditionally, considering them extensions of themselves and committing to their well-being. Children reciprocate this love as they identify their roots and the care provided by their parents. This bond is reinforced over time and through shared experiences. It's anchored in a common lineage and a sense of belonging, which provides a sturdy foundation for love and friendship within the familial unit.

Comradeship: The friendship among comrades, whether they are siblings or close friends, is characterized by shared upbringing, comparable age, and profound connections. Siblings, for instance, often form enduring bonds due to their shared experiences and familial ties. They share their triumphs and tribulations, provide support to one another, and cultivate a sense of camaraderie. This type of friendship is distinguished by a deep understanding, trust, and a mutual sense of belonging.

Spousal Relationship: The bond between spouses is a unique amalgamation of love, friendship, and partnership. It transcends mere companionship to incorporate a deep emotional connection, shared objectives, and a pledge to provide support and care for one another. The love between spouses is predicated on mutual respect, admiration, and an appreciation of each other's strengths. It's a friendship that combines both utility and pleasure, as partners provide mutual support across different facets of life and derive satisfaction from their companionship.

Friendships of Association: Friendships that form within communities, such as among fellow citizens, tribesmen, or colleagues, often stem from shared interests, objectives, or experiences. These friendships may center around a common purpose or shared activities. Although they may not possess the same depth as familial or spousal relationships, they nonetheless offer a sense of belonging, support, and companionship. They're rooted in mutual cooperation, understanding, and a readiness to contribute to the collective well-being.

Acknowledging the unique dynamics inherent in each of

these relationships and the particular nature of love and friendship they embody can enhance our appreciation of the connections we maintain. Love and friendship, whether found within families, among comrades, or in spousal relationships, offer joy, support, and a sense of belonging. They demand mutual understanding, trust, and care to thrive. By embracing and nurturing these relationships, we enrich our lives and cultivate a profound sense of love and happiness.

Chapter 5

Cultivating and Developing Love

5.1 Developing Love in Different Forms of Friendship: A Guide

Love is indeed an integral part of friendship, but its expression varies across different types of friendships. By examining these variations and considering common concerns, we can enhance our understanding and foster love within our relationships.

In friendships of virtue, which involve equals bonding over shared virtues, love is characterized by mutual respect and support. Both individuals aspire to benefit each other, propelled by their shared moral standards. They do not primarily focus on personal gain, but rather rejoice in each other's achievements and find happiness in their friend's growth. Complaints tend to be infrequent in such friendships, given the genuine care and respect shared between equals that facilitate harmonious relations.

In friendships of pleasure, love flourishes through shared experiences and mutual enjoyment. Friends derive joy from each other's company, participating in activities that bring mutual happiness. Their love is grounded in the delight they experience in each other's company. As long as this shared enjoyment persists, complaints are unlikely to arise, as both parties prioritize the mutual joy derived from their interactions.

Friendships of utility pose a distinctive challenge in cultivating love due to their inherently transactional nature. These friendships revolve around mutual benefits and self-interest. To infuse love into them, it's crucial to strike a balance between personal gain and genuine care for the other party. By fostering empathy and endeavoring to understand our friends' needs and desires, we can surpass the purely transactional aspects of these relationships. Addressing complaints in utility-based friendships requires transparent and sincere communication, focusing on reaching fair solutions that accommodate both parties' needs.

To enhance our capacity for love within friendships, it's vital to acknowledge the unique characteristics of each friendship type and approach them consciously. Cherishing the virtues and values that underpin friendships of virtue allows us to develop deeper connections. In friendships of pleasure, maintaining focus on shared experiences and prioritizing mutual happiness can solidify the bond of love. Within friendships of utility, the key lies in harmonizing self-interest with genuine concern, ensuring the relationship transcends mere transactional interactions.

By nurturing empathy, encouraging open communication, and demonstrating a willingness to understand and address concerns, we can mitigate challenges and reinforce the love within our friendships. Love is fostered through acts of kindness, support, and genuine concern for our friends' well-being. When love thrives within our relationships, it serves as a catalyst for personal growth, happiness, and the establishment of enduring bonds.

5.2 Cultivating Mutual Appreciation:
A Key to Enduring Love and Friendship

Love and friendship indeed manifest differently when there exists a disparity of power, status, or capability between the individuals involved. Recognizing and effectively managing these dynamics is essential in maintaining harmony and cultivating love within these relationships.

In such friendships, where one individual holds a superior position—perhaps in terms of virtues, abilities, or resources—expectations can indeed differ. The superior party, recognizing their elevated position, may naturally expect more from the friendship, considering their higher contribution or influence. They may perceive that their superior status or contribution should be reciprocated with more profound respect, appreciation, or other benefits.

Conversely, the individual in an inferior position might experience feelings of inadequacy or dependence. They may yearn for more support, guidance, or resources from their superior friend, creating a certain level of expectation from their end. This situation sets up a dynamic where both parties have distinct expectations that, if not addressed appropriately, can lead to misunderstanding, dissatisfaction, and potential conflict.

Managing these dynamics requires understanding, empathy, and a balance that fosters mutual respect and love. The superior individual, while reasonably expecting recognition and respect for their virtues or contributions, should also be empathetic towards the needs and limitations of the 'inferior' friend. They should aim to offer understanding, compassion, and practical support that can help bridge the gap created by the imbalance.

Similarly, the individual in the 'inferior' position should also make efforts to acknowledge and appreciate the superior friend's value and strengths. They should express gratitude and respect for the superior friend's contributions, which can cultivate mutual appreciation and love. By understanding and valuing each other's unique qualities, an environment of unity can be fostered despite the disparity.

The principle of reciprocity should be at the heart of such friendships. While the nature of contributions might differ based on the friends' status or capabilities, both parties should aim to contribute within their means. The superior friend can offer guidance, mentorship, and resources, while the 'inferior' friend can reciprocate with loyalty, respect, and kindness.

By nurturing mutual respect, understanding, and gratitude, love can thrive even in friendships where there are inherent disparities. By accepting each other's strengths and limitations and finding a common ground for mutual support and appreciation, these friendships can develop strong, lasting bonds. Ultimately, fostering empathy, practicing reciprocity, and demonstrating a genuine desire to uplift and honor each other can allow love to grow and flourish within these unique friendships.

Chapter 6

Love and Friendship

6.1 The Journey of Love and Friendship: A Lifelong Expedition

Friendship indeed plays a vital role in our societal and personal lives. Its value extends beyond mere companionship, fostering social cohesion and, in many respects, supplanting the need for strict justice. Lawmakers and social philosophers often recognize the significance of friendship and prioritize fostering unity and social harmony, akin to the principles of friendship, over strict adherence to justice. In a well-knit society, unity and camaraderie promote social harmony and counteract divisive factions. The existence of genuine friendships can lessen the need for strict justice as friends often treat each other fairly, guided by the principles of mutual respect and understanding. Conversely, in our quest for justice, we often turn to our friends for companionship and support, suggesting an intimate interplay between friendship and justice.

The nobility of friendship is universally recognized. There is an innate admiration for those who show love and affection towards their friends, and individuals with numerous friends are often held in high regard. It's frequently observed that individuals of virtuous nature are more likely to form genuine friendships.

However, the concept of friendship is multifaceted and subject to different interpretations. Some subscribe to the notion that friendship is largely based on similarity, positing that people with similar traits or interests are more likely to form strong bonds. This perspective is encapsulated in aphorisms like "birds of a feather flock together" or "like attracts like". Conversely, others suggest that individuals pursuing similar paths may not necessarily agree or harmonize, reflected in sayings such as "two of a trade never agree".

Numerous theories explore the deeper roots and nuanced elements of friendship. For instance, some theories draw parallels with physical phenomena, such as parched earth seeking rain, or suggest that opposing forces can result in mutual benefit. These varied perspectives underline the complexity of friendship as a human experience that is deeply entwined with character and emotions.

These theories and perspectives prompt us to probe deeper into the nature of friendship. They raise intriguing questions such as whether any two individuals can form a friendship, or whether individuals with wicked tendencies can genuinely forge lasting friendships. It also brings into consideration whether friendship is a single, overarching concept or whether there exist different types of friendship. While some argue for a single continuum of friendship, others note that even different species can exhibit various forms of friendship.

These intricate nuances of friendship have been explored in depth in previous discussions, and revisiting those insights can further our understanding of friendship's complex nature and its integral role in human life.

6.2 Intersections of Affection:

The Profound Bond of Love and Friendship

Across the broad expanse of human history, societies, and cultures, love and friendship stand as universal constants. They serve as essential threads in the fabric of human interaction, binding us together in shared understanding and experience. These constructs, intricate and multi-layered, assume diverse forms within the spectrum of human relationships, often intertwining in ways that enrich and deepen our connection to one another.

Love, with its myriad expressions, can manifest as the indelible bond between family members, the passionate affection found in romantic partnerships, or the profound respect and care that mark some friendships. Each form of love, unique in its characteristics and manifestations, adds a distinctive hue to the human emotional palette, enhancing our capacity for connection and empathy.

Friendship, in parallel, involves elements of mutual understanding, shared experiences, trust, and a sense of belonging. Friendships form an intricate network of bonds that hold us together, anchoring us in times of adversity and celebrating with us in moments of joy. The value of a friendship lies in its capacity to unite individuals in a bond that goes beyond mere utility or transient pleasure, creating a space for genuine connection.

While love and friendship each hold unique spaces within human relationships, there are intersections where they meld into a hybrid form of connection that transcends traditional classifications. In some close relationships, the depth of love can intensify the bond of friendship, adding layers of affection, care, and empathy. Similarly, friendship can foster a distinctive kind of love, one not bound by familial ties or romantic entanglement, but rooted in shared experiences, understanding, and respect.

These bonds, resplendent in their complexity and emotional depth, form the core of human interaction. They encapsulate shared experiences, mutual support, and a joint journey through the diverse landscapes of life. Love and friendship offer humans a sense of companionship and belonging, fostering personal growth, resilience, and shared joy. They create a support network that bolsters us against life's challenges and shares in our triumphs.

However, these bonds are not without their complications. Love and friendship can sometimes give rise to pain, conflict, and discord. Yet, even these challenges provide opportunities for personal growth, emotional maturity, and a deepening of empathy and understanding. As such, despite the occasional turmoil, love and friendship remain indispensable facets of the human experience, fostering an innate sense of connection and shared journey that is integral to our collective and individual narratives.

Conclusion

In "The Power and Beauty of Friendship," we embarked on an in-depth exploration of the complexities and nuances of love and friendship. We analyzed the genesis of bonds, shedding light on the distinctive types of friendships, their roots in companionship, and the power they hold. The dynamics of friendships, including the beauty found in unequal friendships, the trifecta of connection, character, and equality, and the subtleties present within these relationships, were thoroughly examined.

The inseparable duo of love and friendship was dissected, highlighting their true nature, the essence of emotional connections they establish, and the harmony of affection and fairness they foster. We dove into the power and influence of love, its manifestation in various relationships, and the role it plays in nurturing growth and development.

Additionally, we provided guidance on fostering love within different forms of friendships, emphasizing the role of mutual appreciation as a crucial ingredient in enduring love and friendships. As we conclude, it's clear that the journey of love and friendship is indeed a lifelong expedition, filled with joy, challenges, growth, and profound experiences.

Throughout the journey, we reaffirm that love and friendship remain the cornerstone of human connection, defining our experiences, shaping our identities, and providing a lens through which we perceive the world. The essence of connection, captured in the dance between love and friendship, is a testament to our shared humanity, our capacity for empathy, and our intrinsic need for communal bonds. As we continue our personal journeys, let us embrace these insights, nourishing the love and friendships that add color, depth, and meaning to our lives.

Bibliography

1. Aristotle - "Nicomachean Ethics" (Penguin Classics; Reissue edition, 2004): A foundational text in Western philosophy, the Nicomachean Ethics offers an extensive discussion on friendship and its various types.

2. C.S. Lewis - "The Four Loves" (HarperOne; Reprint edition, 2017): In this book, C.S. Lewis explores the nature of love from a Christian and philosophical perspective, including affection, friendship, eros, and charity.

3. Shasta Nelson - "Frientimacy: How to Deepen Friendships for Lifelong Health and Happiness" (Seal Press, 2016): This book offers insights on developing deeper connections in friendships.

4. Dale Carnegie - "How to Win Friends and Influence People" (Pocket Books; Reissue edition, 1998): While it's not solely about friendship, Carnegie's book offers valuable advice on interpersonal relationships.

5. Robin Dunbar - "Friends: Understanding the Power of our Most Important Relationships" (Little, Brown Spark, 2021): Dunbar presents a mix of scientific research and human stories to highlight the importance of friendships in our lives.

6. bell hooks - "All About Love: New Visions" (William Morrow Paperbacks; 1st edition, 2001): This book delves into

the nature of love, its various forms, and its intersection with our lives and relationships.

6. Plato - "Lysis" or "On Friendship" (CreateSpace Independent Publishing Platform, 2016): In this dialogue written by Plato, Socrates discusses the nature of friendship with two young boys.

7. Plato - "Symposium" (Penguin Classics; Revised edition, 2003): This classic piece of literature involves Socrates and others engaged in a discussion about the nature of love during a banquet. Socrates' speech, in particular, examines the concept of love from a philosophical standpoint.

www.ingramcontent.com/pod-product-compliance
Lightning Source LLC
Chambersburg PA
CBHW022052190326
41520CB00008B/781